SPATIAL DISORIENTATION FOR DIVERS

By: AJ Powell

15 January 2022

Table of Contents

Preface	6
Introduction	8
Types of Spatial Disorientation	10
Understanding Equilibrium and Movement	12
Sensory Systems	14
Sensory Illusions	32
Stress and Fatigue in Diving	46
Prevention of Spatial Disorientation	56
Treatment of Spatial Disorientation	64
Appendix	70

Spatial Disorientation for Divers
AJ Powell (USA, Ret.)
Copyright © 2022
All rights reserved.

All diving images within this publication are original images taken by and owned by AJ Powell, and copyright © is retained by the owner.

This publication is intended for educational purposes. Information contained within this publication has been reproduced from original sources, including Aeromedical Training for Flight Personnel. Distribution of these sources has been approved for public release and is unlimited in nature, and access for free use of these sources is listed as public domain. All medical information contained herein is accurate to original sources, unaltered, and application to diving operations may be easily referenced and verifiable per original sources. All effort has been made to retain consistency, applicability, and authenticity to original sources and their direct applicability to diving operations and safety.

What would you interpret about the environment in the image below? How do you know what is near and what is far? What do you see that can help you determine which way is up, where the horizontal plane is situated, and whether or not the diver is correctly orientated to it?

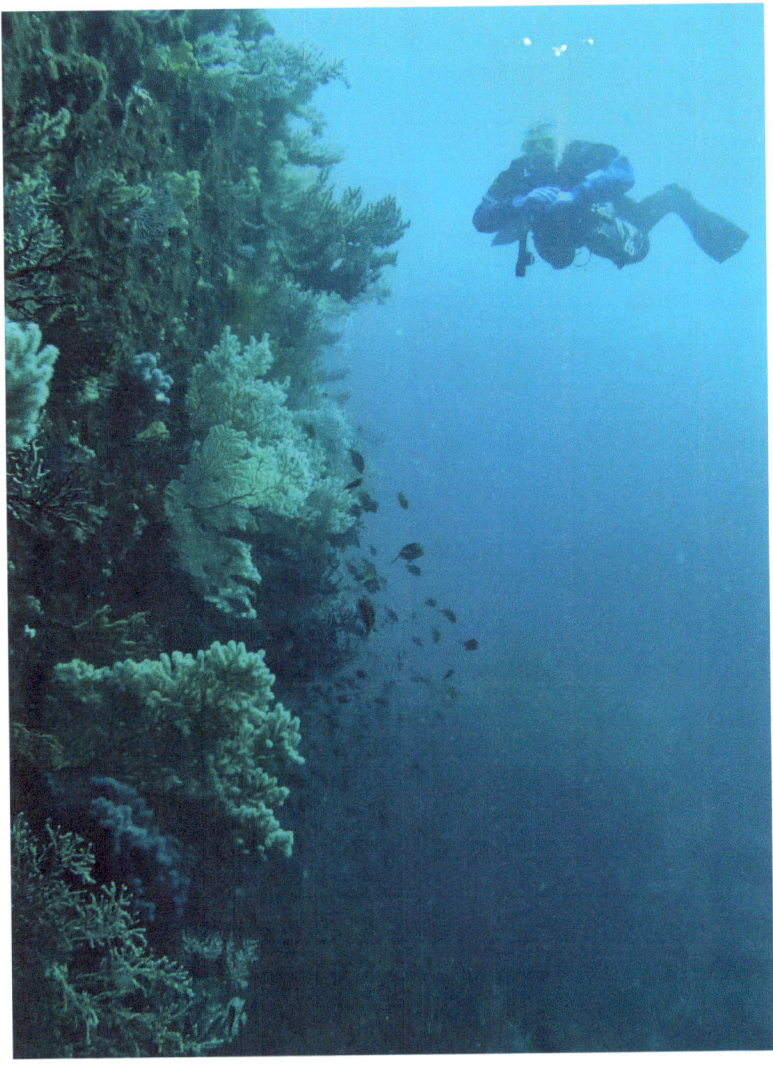

PREFACE

Human beings are physiologically designed to use our senses to orient ourselves within the environment we inhabit while standing on the ground. Our brain interprets what we see and feel to produce unconscious and intuitive corrective actions in order to maintain proper balance and orientation along the X, Y, and Z axis. While sight makes up the largest sensory input contributing to our spatial orientation (We are "visual" creatures), our middle ear (semicircular canals) combined with the inertial movement of our organs within the body, contribute greatly to our ability to interpret correctly what is happening to our bodies in relation to the space we inhabit.

However, whenever we are removed from direct contact with the ground (or a stabilizing hold)—e.g. flying through the air or diving underwater—we are physiologically susceptible to a large number of visual, vestibular (middle ear), and proprioceptive (pressure and organs) illusions that confuse and can even incapacitate our brain's ability to correctly interpret what is happening, causing us to become spatially disorientated. Spatial disorientation can have side effects ranging from minor illusions or mistakes, to completely incapacitating physiological effects that can result in unconsciousness, injury, or death.

This publication was written to address the lack of information that exists today regarding spatial disorientation and its effects as it relates to divers. Most divers already maintain some degree of understanding that spatial disorientation exists due to feeling the effects of disorientating sensory illusions on nearly every dive. However, while they may know they experienced "something" for a brief period of time, they may not know what it was, the mechanisms that caused it, or how to deal with it. This is largely contributable to the absence of inclusion of spatial disorientation throughout courses and educational materials, and awareness training and lectures, that are a part of every divers progression. Yet it is found in one place consistently, as a common source contributing factor to dive incidents and accidents.

Spatial disorientation is a root factor from which an array of other emergencies stem. It causes divers to choose the wrong direction to proceed, to dive deeper than they should, to surface prematurely, to get confused and lost, to panic, to make a series of decisions based on wrong information that leads to an accident, and more. It can trick you into thinking nothing is wrong, or believing something is when no problem exists, and it can make you nauseous, dizzy, cause seizures, or give you such an overwhelming sensation of movement that you black out and go unconscious—though extraordinarily rare.

Divers, therefore, should be well-educated on the subject of spatial disorientation, its effects, sensory illusions, stress, and prevention and recovery methods, and this publication will attempt to provide that information. Divers that understand what spatial disorientation is are more likely to recognize it when encountered, and more likely to make the right decisions that could prevent a mishap.

INTRODUCTION

Spatial disorientation contributes more to causing accidents than any other psychological problem in a multi-directional space, such as diving underwater or flying through the air. Regardless of their amount of time or experience underwater, all divers are subject to disorientation. The human body is structured to perceive changes in movement when standing vertically on land in relation to the surface of the earth. When diving, the human sensory systems—the visual system, vestibular system, and proprioceptive system—can and will give the brain erroneous orientation information due to positioning and movement of the body in a space and along an axis foreign to our biological design. This information can and will cause some degree of sensory illusions, which in-turn lead to spatial disorientation, that further leads to confusion, lost time in actions, potentially harmful or dangerous reactions, and a developing spiral of out-of-control events leading to an accident or death.

What is "Spatial Disorientation"?

Spatial disorientation (Spatial D.) is an individual's inability to determine his or her position, attitude, and motion relative to the space they are occupying and/or any significant objects within visual range; for example, large rocks, down lines, artificial structures, the surface, the bottom, a boat, etc. When Spatial D. occurs, divers are unable to see, believe, interpret, or mentally prove the information derived from their instruments (computer, depth gauge, compass, etc.). Instead, they have a strong tendency to rely on the false information that their senses provide, or the sensory input becomes so strong that it can cause panic, confusion, and even incapacitation.

Why is Spatial Disorientation Important for Divers?

Understanding the human sensory organs, the mechanisms for spatial disorientation to occur, and how it affects the senses, allows you to recognize when you are experiencing sensory illusions, and the ability to recover from those disorientating effects. Nearly every diver has likely encountered some form of spatial disorientation to some degree on almost every dive, yet most couldn't tell you what they felt or why. Worse, when divers do encounter some degree of disorientation caused by sensory illusions, many could not tell you how to recover. Since spatial disorientation is a root factor that directly and indirectly contributes to dive accidents, it is imperative for every diver to maintain even a basic understanding of its causes, effects, and prevention and recovery methods. Therefore, inclusion of spatial disorientation information as a core component of a divers training progression at every level is the keystone to prevention, and will result in a safer, more aware, and better trained diver.

TYPES OF SPATIAL DISORIENTATION

Type I (Unrecognized): A disoriented diver does not perceive any indication of spatial disorientation. In other words, he or she does not think anything is wrong. What the diver sees—or thinks they see—is corroborated by other senses.

Type I disorientation is the most dangerous type because the diver—completely unaware of any problem—fails to recognize that a problem exists, and is unable to make any corrections. Unfortunately, this type of disorientation is the most common encountered by most divers. Yet fortunately, the majority of sensory illusions most divers encounter are minor, and easily corrected. In fact, most divers work through Type I disorientation without knowing it. However, this type still has the potential to result in fatal mishaps due to the diver believing everything is fine until it is too late, which is why it is the most dangerous.

In the case of Type I disorientation, the diver may see instruments functioning properly, so there is no suspicion of any malfunctions. Further, there may be no indication of any equipment malfunctions, so the diver may perceive everything is performing normally. As such, the diver fails to recognize an error exists and carries on, believing what they "feel", and often not verifying that against the information their instruments provide.

An example of this type of spatial disorientation would be the "height/depth perception illusion" whereby, in an open area with a clear view of a white sandy bottom, and no other obvious objects, the diver descends too quickly to the bottom and ends up hitting the bottom, because a lack of other visual cues caused the diver to lose depth perception. Without any other objects to make a determination on how far away the bottom actually is, their misinterpretation led them to believe it was further way than it actually was, resulting in plummeting into it.

Type II (Recognized): A disorientated diver perceives a problem exists, however, may or may not recognize it as spatial disorientation. They may feel that what they see and feel from sensory input is "off", or recognize they could be suffering from symptoms of one or more sensory illusions, however, may not use instruments or environmental cues to fully understand the problem and take corrective actions.

Type III (Incapacitating): A diver experiences spatial disorientation—such as one or more sensory illusions—of such an overwhelming sensation of movement that he or she cannot orient themselves by using visual cues or instruments. The diver might remain conscious, however, will be unable to take any major corrective actions to stop the sensory illusion from occurring. In this case, the event may not be fatal so long as the diver can remain calm and in place until the sensation is over or lessened enough for them to begin ascent. Or, though extremely rare, the diver may be rendered unconscious, in which case, survivability is less likely.

UNDERSTANDING EQUILIBRIUM AND MOVEMENT

Three sensory systems—the visual, vestibular, and proprioceptive systems—are especially important in maintaining equilibrium and balance. Normally, the combined functioning of these senses maintains equilibrium and prevents spatial disorientation. However, while diving, the visual system is considered the most reliable of the three. In the absence of vision, the vestibular and proprioceptive systems are unreliable for orientation in the water.

Try this sometime: Technical divers, military divers, and even cave divers must perform skills underwater without the use of vision during training. During these events, it is often the case that most report no ability to tell their attitude and trim, nor their stability of depth (buoyancy). They can't tell if they are horizontal or pitched slightly to one side, they can't tell their position in relation to other nearby objects, and the only way they know if they are ascending or descending is when they feel/hear pressure escaping from the middle ear and sinus or feel a squeeze. The next time you go diving with a buddy, find a nearby object and adjust to perfect neutral buoyancy. Then take turns removing your mask, and trying to stay exactly in the same position, attitude, and depth in relation to the object for a minute, with your buddy watching for safety. Then put your mask back on, clear, and see if you could stay put or if you moved. Few divers out there have an intuitive ability to stay put, while most take years to develop this skill. The ability to stay put when you can't see is the ability to accurately understand and correctly interpret sensory input from the vestibular and proprioceptive systems. Because few people can do this naturally, it is often the case these systems are considered unreliable for correct orientation by themselves, but they will cause a variety of illusions easily that can disorientate or even incapacitate.

Human beings can sense physical motion through space in 12 different positional changes. These include: Forward, Backward, Left, Right, Up, Down, Rotation Right, Rotation Left, Tilt Up, Tilt Down, Yaw Right, and Yaw Left. As momentum is felt in relation to any of these positional changes, the visual, vestibular, and proprioceptive systems sense changes in monocular cues, acceleration, and gravity, to work together to orient and balance the body.

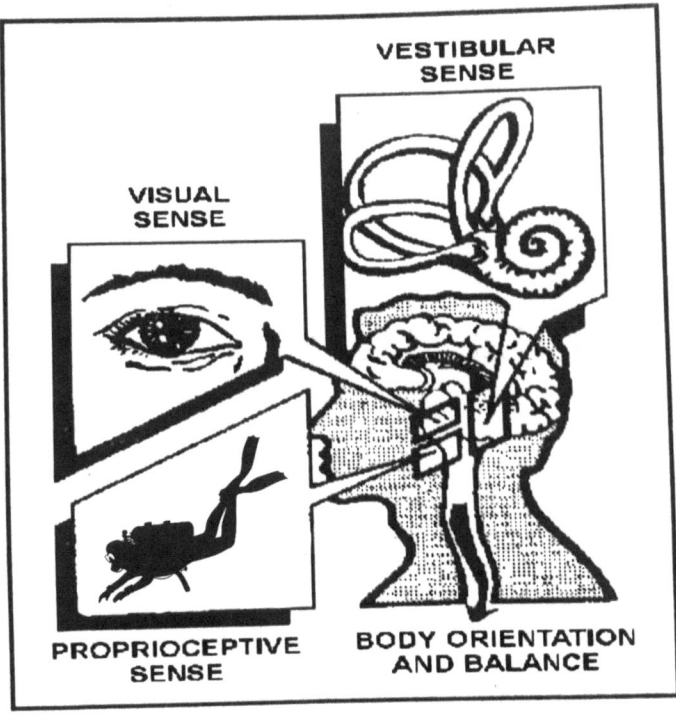

SENSORY SYSTEMS

Visual system

Of the three sensory systems, the visual system is the most important in maintaining equilibrium and orientation. Human beings are "visual creatures" and roughly between 70% to 80% of our total sensory input is visual. to some extent, the eyes can help determine motion, speed, direction, and orientation by comparing the position of yourself relative to some other object or point of reference.

On open ocean dives, and night dives in open water, divers may not have any fixed points of reference by which to orientate themselves. Instead, they must rely on visual sensory input from their instruments and environmental factors (like bubbles if diving open circuit) to aid in spatial orientation. The decision and ability to rely on the visual sense, and use effectively instruments rather than what a diver "feels" from their other senses, demands disciplined training.

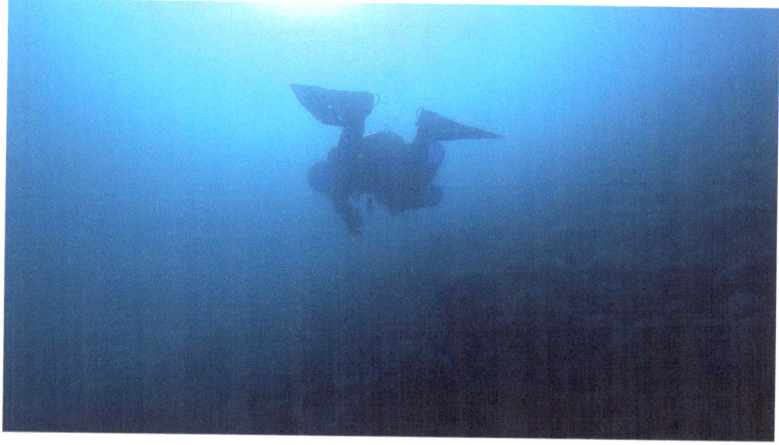

Since divers rely more on the visual sense than any other sense, it's important for divers to understand that good depth perception, and good visual acuity, are directly contributable visual factors to a diver's performance underwater. Although vision is the most accurate and reliable sense, visual cues can be misleading, contributing to incidents and accidents. Divers should therefore be aware of the basics of how the eyes and vision works in order to recognize disorientating illusions when encountered.

Visual Deficiencies

One contributing factor associated in safe diving is that divers should be able to recognize and understand common visual deficiencies. Important eye problems related to the degraded visual acuity and depth perception include myopia, hyperopia, astigmatism, presbyopia, and retinal rivalry.

Myopia - This condition, often referred to as near-sightedness, is caused by an error in refraction in which the lens of the eye does not focus an image directly onto the retina. When a myopic person views an image at a distance, the actual focal point of the eye is in front of the retinal plane (wall), causing blurred vision. Thus, distant objects are not seen clearly; only nearby objects are in focus.

Night Myopia - At night, and in deeper depths underwater—even during the day—blue wavelengths of light prevail in the visible portion of the spectrum. Therefore, slightly nearsighted (myopic) individuals may experience blurred vision. Even individuals with perfect vision will find that sharpness and clarity of

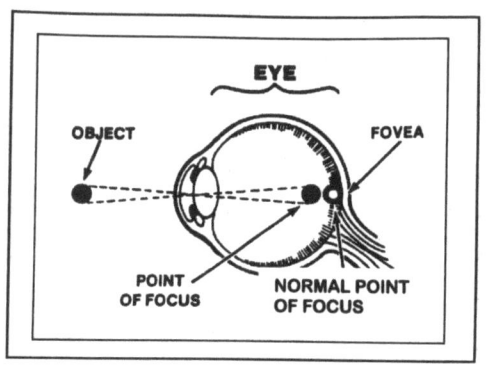

vision decreases as pupil diameter increases. For individuals with mild refractive errors, these factors combine to make vision unacceptably blurred unless they have a corrective lens mask.

Hyperopia - Also caused by an error in refraction — the lens of the eye does not focus an image directly on the retina — this condition is often called farsightedness. When a hyperopic individual looks at a nearby object, the actual focal point of the eye is behind the retinal plane, causing blurred vision. Objects that are nearby are not seen clearly; only more distant objects are in focus.

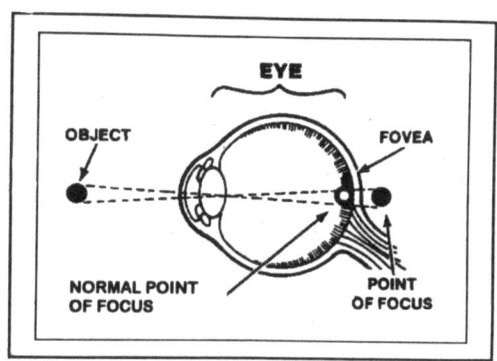

Astigmatism - This is an unequal curvature of the cornea or lens of the eye. A ray of light is spread over a diffused area in one meridian. In normal vision, light is sharply focused on the retina. Astigmatism is the inability to focus different meridians simultaneously.

Presbyopia - This condition is part of the normal aging process, which causes the lens of the eye to harden. Beginning in the early teens, the human eye gradually loses the ability to accommodate for and focus on nearby objects. When people are about 40 years old, their eyes are unable to focus at normal reading distances without reading glasses. Reduced illumination interferes with focus depth of the lens (cataract formation). Divers with early cataracts may have difficulty seeing instruments under bright light conditions. This problem is due to the light scattering as it enters the eye. This glare sensitivity can be disabling under certain circumstances. Glare disability, related to contrast sensitivity, is the inability to detect objects against varying shades of backgrounds. Other visual functions that decline with age and that affect performance include: dynamic acuity, recovery from glare, function under low illumination, and information processing.

Retinal Rivalry - Eyes may experience this problem when attempting to simultaneously perceive two dissimilar objects independently. This phenomenon may occur when CCR divers view objects while one eye has a HUD positioned in front of it. If one eye views the image on the HUD, while the other is scanning in front of the diver, a conflict arises within the total perception of the diver. Quite often, the dominant eye will override the non-dominant eye, causing the diver to possibly miss information delivered to the non-dominant eye. Additionally, this rivalry may lead to ciliary spasms, eye pain, and headaches. Mental conditioning and practice may appear to alleviate this condition, but it is not always the case that the condition can be prevented.

Anatomy and Physiology of the Eye

Visual acuity is the eye's ability to resolve spatial detail. Normal visual acuity is 20/20. A value of 20/80 indicates that an individual reads at 20 feet the letters and numbers that an individual with normal acuity reads at 80 feet away. The human eye functions like a camera. It has an instantaneous field of view, which is oval and typically measures 120 degrees vertically by 150 degrees horizontally. When two eyes are used for viewing, the overall FoV measures about 120 degrees vertically by 200 degrees horizontally.

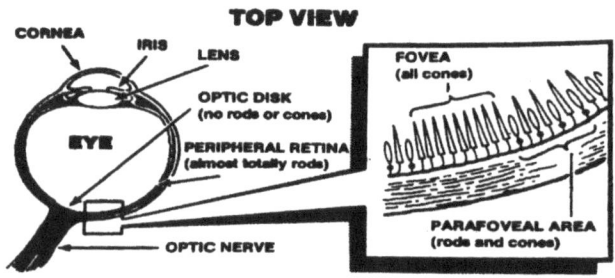

As light enters the eye and passes through the pupil and the lens, it is directed upon the retina. The retina is a complex, structured membrane, consisting of 10 layers, called the Jacob's membrane, and that contains many tiny photoreceptors cells, called rods and cones. When light stimulates the retina, it produces a chemical change within these cells that send nerve impulses to the brain via the optic nerve. The brain deciphers the impulses and creates a mental image that interprets what the individual is viewing.

Vision is possible because of the chemical reactions within the eye. The chemical iodopsin is always present within the cone cells. Iodopsin permits the cone cells to respond immediately to visual stimulation, regardless of the level of ambient light. However, rod cells contain an extremely light-sensitive chemical called rhodopsin, more commonly referred to as visual purple. Rhodopsin is not always present in the rods because light bleaches it out and renders the rods inactive to stimulation. Rhodopsin is so sensitive that light exposure can bleach out all visual purple within seconds.

For night vision to take place, rhodopsin must build up in the rods. The average time required to gain the greatest sensitivity is between 30 to 45 minutes in a dark environment. When fully sensitized (dark adapted), the rod cells may become up to 10,000 times more sensitive than at the start of the dark adaptation period. Through a dilated pupil, total light sensitivity may increase in the human eye 100,000 times.

Types of Vision

The three types of vision are photopic, mesopic, and scotopic, and each type requires different sensory stimuli or ambient lighting conditions.

Photopic Vision - This is the type of vision humans experience during daylight or under high levels of artificial illumination, such as diving at night, in a wreck, or in a cave, while using underwater lights. The cones concentrated in the fovea centralis of the retina are primarily responsible for vision in bright light. Because of the high-level light condition, rod cells are bleached out and become less effective. Sharp image interpretation and color vision are characteristics of photopic vision, and the fovea centralis is automatically directed toward an object by a visual fixation reflex. Therefore, under photopic conditions, the eye uses central vision for interpretation, especially for determining details.

Mesopic Vision - This is the type of vision humans experience at dawn and dusk, or under full moonlight and lower daytime lighting conditions underwater, for example, when diving deeper than 60ft (18m). Vision is achieved by a combination of rods and cones, and visual acuity steadily decreases with declining light. Color vision is reduced (degraded) as the light level decreases, and the cones become less effective. Mesopic vision is the most dangerous of all three types of vision for divers with regards to spatial disorientation, because it is the point at which the greatest number of visual illusions are possible.

Scotopic Vision - This is the type of vision humans experience under low-light level environments such as partial moonlight and starlight conditions, very dimly lit rooms, and deep and/or confined diving environments with little ambient light. Cones become ineffective, causing poor resolution of detail, and visual acuity decreases to 20/200 or less. Additionally, all color perception is lost as rods only allow for grey vision (black and white and shades of gray). A central blind spot (night blind spot) occurs when cone-cell sensitivity is completely lost, and peripheral vision is the primary vision used for viewing with scotopic vision.

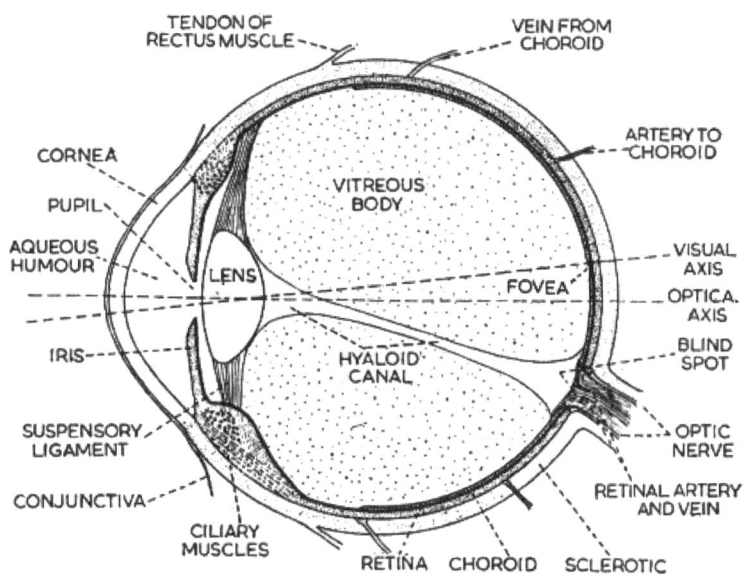

Monocular Cues

The cues to distance estimation and depth perception are easy to recognize when central vision is used under good illumination. When light hits the retina, signals are sent to the brain and translated into the image of the world we see. We use this information to orientate ourselves physically according to the horizontal plane. Monocular cues are how we accomplish this, and they allow us to interpret our position relative to everything else around us. Everything from the size of objects, the location of objects, their relation to each other, their relation to the horizon, their motion in relation to us and each other, and more, are all cues we use to determine their true size, distance, and direction in relation to ourselves. As light levels decrease, the ability to judge distance accurately degrades and the eyes are vulnerable to illusions.

Memory aid for monocular cues: **GRAM**

Geometric Perspective

Objects may appear to have a different shape when viewed at varying distances and from different angles. Memory aid: LAV

Linear Perspective - Parallel lines (pipelines, cables, trenches, etc.) converge as distance away from the observer increases.

Apparent Foreshortening - The true shape of an object or feature appears elliptical when viewed from a distance. As the distance to the object or feature decreases, the apparent perspective changes to its true shape or form.

<u>Vertical Position on the Field</u> - Objects farther away appear higher on the horizon than closer objects.

Retinal Image Size

The physical size of the object as it hits the retina is interpreted by the brain to be "a certain size" based on known cues about the object. Memory aid: KITO

<u>Known Size of Objects</u> - The closer the object is, the larger its size on the retina will be. By experience, the brain learns to estimate the distance of familiar objects by the size of their retinal image. A structure projects a specific angle on the retina, based on its distance from the observer. If the angle is small, the observer judges the structure to be at a great distance. A larger angle indicates to the observer that the structure is close. To use this cue, the observer must know or have a good idea of the actual size of the object, and have some degree of prior visual experience with it. If no experience exists, our brain tends to gravitate toward using motion parallax to determine distance.

<u>Increasing/Decreasing Size of Objects</u> - If an object's size appears to be increasing, the object is getting closer. If the object's size is constant, the object is at a fixed distance.

<u>Terrestrial Association</u> - Objects associated together are typically judged to be at the same distance (guilty by association). Comparison of one object, such as

another diver, with another object of a known size, such as a boulder, will help to determine the relative size and apparent distance of the object from the observer.

<u>Overlapping Contours</u> - Overlapped objects are further away.

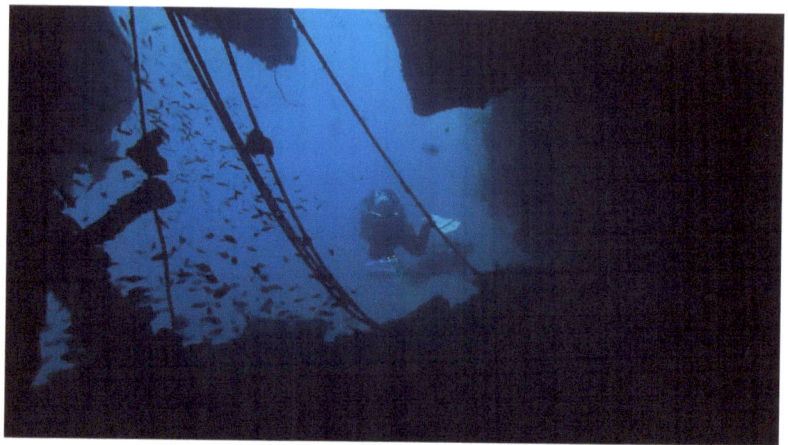

Aerial Perspective

The clarity of, and the shadow cast, by an object are perceived by the brain, and are used as cues for estimating distances. Memory aid: FLL

<u>Fading of Colors</u> - Objects viewed through dust, sand, haze, etc., are seen less distinctly and appear to be at a greater distance than they actually are. If atmospheric transmission of light is unrestricted, an object is seen more distinctly and appears to be closer than it actually is.

Loss of Detail - Objects have less detail the further away they are. Environmental factors increase the effects of degraded texture and detail of objects throughout the visual field. This loss of details, in turn, severely decreases depth perception and is a contributing factor in relation to misjudgments of what is seen or not seen and the occurrence of incidents related to the misjudgments.

Position of Light Source - Every object will cast a shadow if there is a light source. If the shadow is toward the observer, the object is closer than the light source.

Motion Parallax

This is often considered the most important visual cue to depth perception. Motion parallax refers to the apparent, relative motion of stationary objects as viewed by an observer who is moving in a given direction. Nearer objects appear to move faster than objects farther away, and objects at a great distance appear to remain stationary. The rate of apparent movement depends on the distance that the observer is from the object. Objects near the diver will appear to move rapidly, while distant objects will seem as if they don't move at all. Thus, objects that appear to be moving rapidly are judged to be nearby, while those moving slowly are judged to be at a greater distance.

Vestibular system

The inner ear contains the vestibular system, which contains the motion and gravity-detecting sensory organs. This system is located in the temporal bone on each side of the head. Each vestibular apparatus consists of two distinct structures: the semicircular canals and the vestibule proper, which contains the otolith organs. Both the semicircular canals and the otolith organs sense changes in attitude, angular acceleration and deceleration, and changes in gravity by pitch.

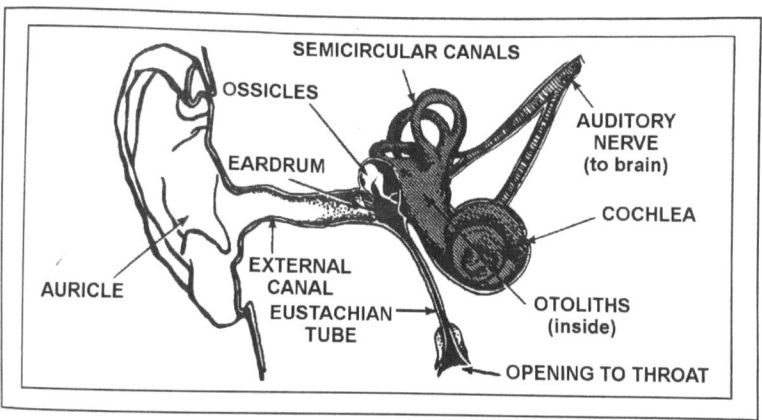

Otolith organs

The otolith organs are small sacs located in the vestibule. Sensory hairs project from each macula into the otolithic membrane, an overlaying gelatinous membrane that contains chalk-like crystals, called otoliths. The otolith organs respond to gravity and linear acceleration/deceleration. Changes in the position of the head, relative to the gravitational force, cause the otolithic member to shift position on the macula. When the sensory hairs bend, it signals a change in the head position.

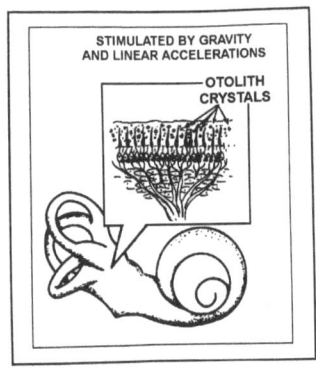 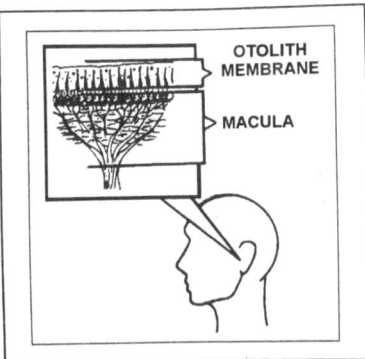

When the head is upright, a "resting" frequency of nerve impulses is generated by the hair cells. When the head is tilted, the "resting" frequency is altered, and the brain is informed of the new position.

Linear accelerations/decelerations also stimulate the otolith organs. The body cannot physically distinguish between the inertial forces resulting from linear accelerations and the forces of gravity. A forward acceleration results in backward displacement of the otolithic membranes. When an adequate visual reference is not available, divers may experience an illusion of backwards tilt.

Semicircular canals

The semicircular canals of the inner ear sense changes in angular acceleration. The canals will react to any changes in pitch, roll, or yaw attitude. They are situated in three planes, perpendicular to each other, and are filled with a fluid called endolymph. The inertial torque resulting from angular acceleration in the plane of the canals puts this fluid into motion. The motion of the fluid bends the cupula, a gelatinous structure located in the ampulla of the canals. This, in turn, moves the hairs of the hair cells situated beneath the cupula. The movement stimulates the vestibular nerve. These nerve impulses are then transmitted to the brain, where they are interpreted as rotation of the head.

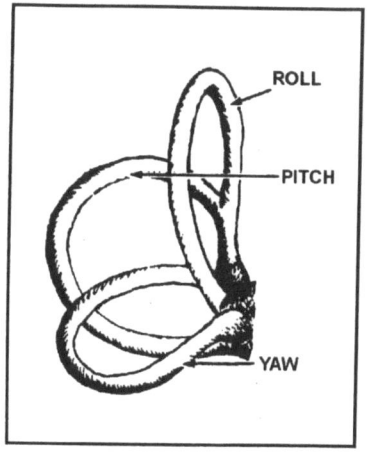

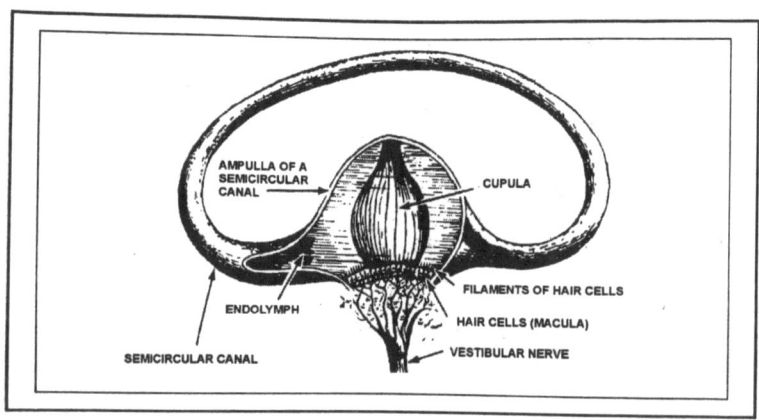

When no acceleration takes place, the hair cells are upright. The body senses that no turn has occurred. When a semicircular canal is put into motion during a rotational acceleration, the fluid within one or more canals lags behind the acceleration. This lag creates a relative counter movement of the fluid within the canal. The canal wall and the cupula move in the opposite direction from the motion of the fluid. The brain interprets the movement of the hairs to be a turn in the same direction as the canal wall, and the body correctly senses that a turn has been made.

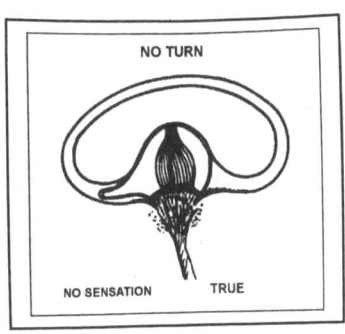 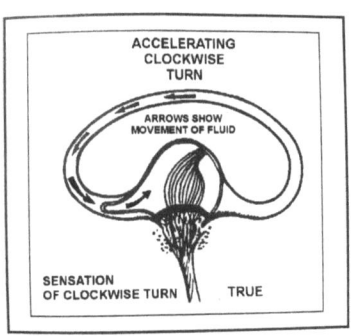

If the turn continues at a constant rate for several seconds longer, the motion of the fluid in the canals catches up with the canal walls. This allows the fluid to stabilize in its current position. With the fluid no longer moving, the hairs are no longer bent, and the brain receives the false impression that the turning has stopped, and the result is a false sensation of no turn occurring. When the rotation slows or stops, the fluid in the canal moves briefly, sending a signal to the brain that is falsely interpreted as body movement in the opposite direction. In an attempt to

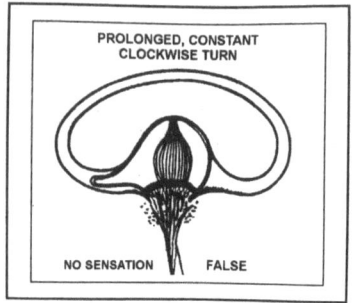 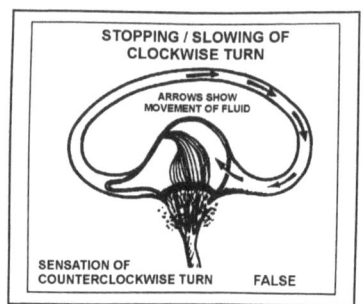

correct the falsely perceived counter turn, the diver may turn back into the original direction as before, resulting in a continuation of the original turn.

Proprioceptive system

The proprioceptive system reacts to the sensation of pressure on joints, muscles, skin, and slight changes in the position of internal organs. It is closely associated with the vestibular system and, to a lesser degree, the visual system. Physical forces act upon the diver in the water, and as the water moves, and the diver's body moves, motion is perceived by the diver as changes in pressure across muscles, joints, and the skin, and movements of the internal organs, sends signals to the brain that are interpreted as movement in the opposite direction.

As the body moves forward, pressure felt across the front area of the body, and rearward movement of the internal organs, gives the sensation of the body moving in a forward direction. As waves push a diver around in one direction and then another, opposite movements between the body and the organs, combined with increasing and decreasing pressures felt across one side and then the other, sends signals to the brain that are interpreted as back and forth movement of the body. If this persists for a prolonged period of time, the brain begins to retain the information in an attempt to stabilize the sensations. After the diver exits the water, false or "ghost sensations" of movement may be continued to be felt by the diver to a period of time.

(After a longer dive, it is common for many divers to still feel the sway of the ocean for a period of time after they get out of the water.)

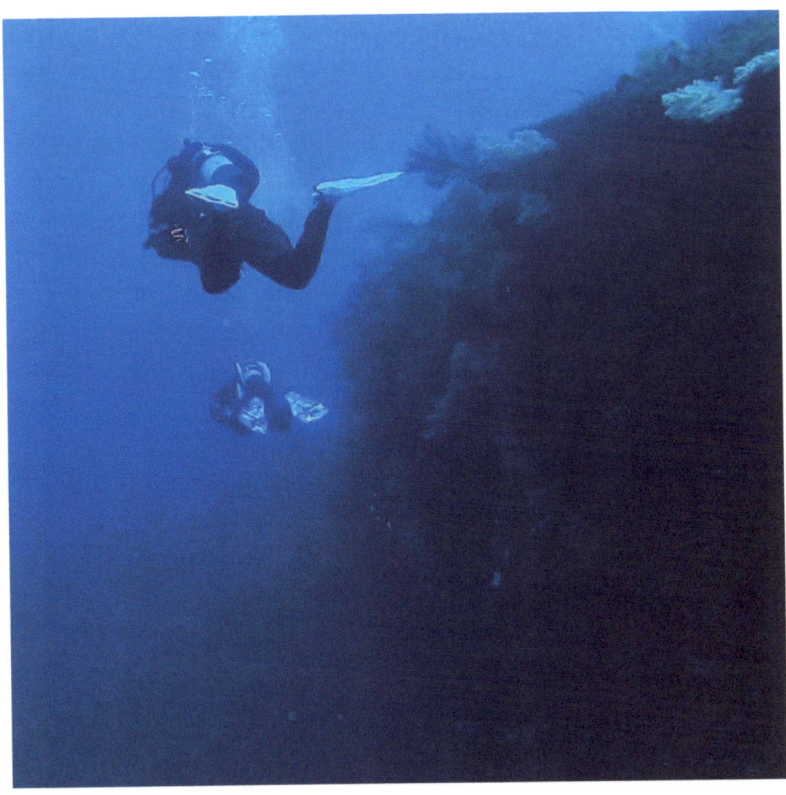

SENSORY ILLUSIONS

Visual Illusions

The visual system isn't perfect, and much of it relies on our past experience. Our brain uses what we already know (or think we know) about everything we see to make determinations regarding our orientation, and any time what we see doesn't match what we think we know or what we're currently feeling in conjunction with the other sensory systems, a conflict exists. This is how visual illusions manifest.

Illusions give false impressions or misconceptions of actual conditions; therefore, divers must understand the types of illusions that can occur and the resulting disorientation. Although the visual system is the most reliable of the senses, some illusions can result from misinterpreting what is seen; what is perceived is not always accurate. Even with the references found in the surrounding environment, and the information provided by instruments, divers must be on guard to interpret information correctly so they can avoid becoming disorientated.

There are 12 visual illusions divers can encounter, and the memory aid for these is:

Fire! Fire! Fire! - CRASH - SAR - L
(FFF-CRASH-SAR-L)

Flicker Vertigo - Light seen through propellers or other rotating devices, or that flickers due to waves at any near constant interval between 4 to 20 flashes per second, can cause nausea, dizziness, and possible convulsions. Viewing a flickering light can be both distracting and annoying for many people, however for some, photic stimuli at certain frequencies can cause nausea, make them feel dizzy, or even very rarely, induce seizures in individuals who are susceptible for flicker-induced epilepsy. Individuals with a past history of flicker-induced epileptic episodes should be especially cautious when diving to not put themselves in a location in the water where light may be flickering through the water from above.

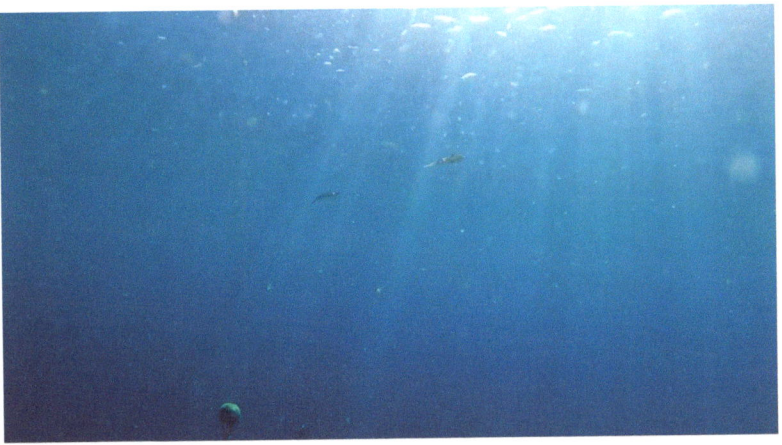

Fascination/Fixation - This can be separated into two categories: Task Saturation and Target Fixation. Task saturation—commonly called "task loading" by many dive agencies—may occur during the accomplishment of even simple tasks while diving. Divers may become overwhelmed by one or more tasks or problems that they lose the ability to manage them effectively. This causes them to become so engrossed with one problem or task that they fail to properly scan their surroundings, and pay attention to the others. Target fixation—commonly called "target hypnosis"—occurs when a diver ignores information and/or cues due to intense focus on one object or goal, resulting in missing other, perhaps more important information or cues that my help them solve the problem or accomplish the task, or to recognize that more important problems or tasks need attention rather than the one they are focused on. An example of this may be a diver focused so intently on performing a gas switch at a targeted depth, that they ignore the fact that they may have either sunk to a deeper depth or blown past their target depth, or failed to recognize assistance.

(A diver focused on taking notes while simultaneously trying to maintain trim, buoyancy, and distance from an object can easily suffer from Fascination/Fixation, causing them to forget about the world around them, and possibly miss more important/critical information such as depth, time, gas consumption, etc.)

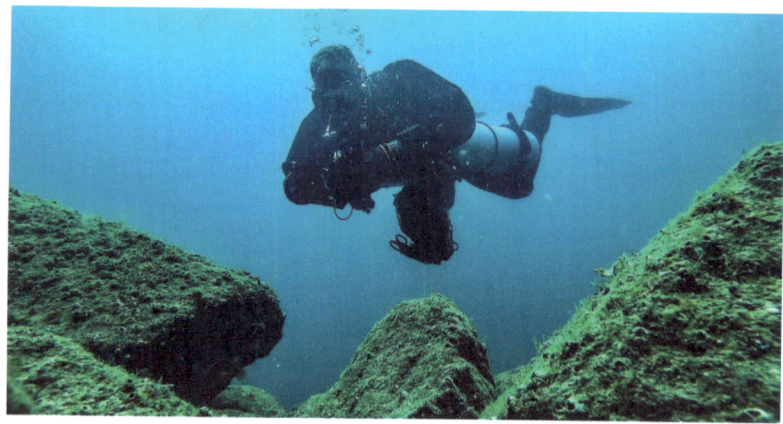

False Horizons - Confusing sand, silt, or dust cloud formations with the horizon or ground. This occurs when a diver confuses the silhouette of large-scale objects or shadows in the distance, or cloud formations with what they believe to be the true horizontal horizon or ground. The illusion occurs when a diver subconsciously chooses the only reference point available for orientation of their body to the horizontal plane. A sloping cloud of silt hanging in the water, or the appearance of a continuous sloping shadow off in the distance, may be difficult to perceive as anything but horizontal if it extends for any great distance in the diver's peripheral vision. Judgement is further impaired due to visual restrictions caused by the diver's mask, which limits the diver's field of view to a certain number of degrees on either side. Divers may perceive the false horizon to be the actual horizontal plane the body naturally aligns to, causing them to alter their trim and assume an attitude even with the new plane of reference. This condition is often insidious and goes undetected until the diver suddenly recognizes it and makes the transition to the true horizontal plane using either instruments or another reference point, and may result in leading to the creation of other, more serious illusions.

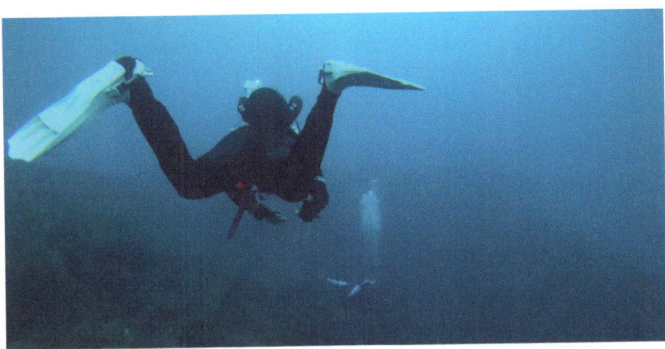

Crater Illusion - Illusion of falling into a crater with up-sloping terrain in all directions. This illusion is typically caused by light distortion seen through the mask when looking straight down on a sunny day around mid-day, while descending in clear water to a large flat bottom, and with no other major objects nearby. The sunlight, also focused straight downward, combined with a lack of other visual cues on the bottom, will combine to create the illusion of descending into a crater or depression, with up-sloping terrain on all sides. This illusionary depression lulls the diver into continuing their descent, resulting in prematurely impacting the bottom, which may or may not pose a hazard to the diver, disturb the environmental conditions, or impact wildlife or the dive site.

Relative Motion - Falsely perceived self-motion in relation to the motion of another object. The most common example of this is when an individual in a car is stopped at a traffic light and another car pulls alongside. The individual that was stopped at the light perceives the forward motion of the second car as their own motion rearward. This results in the individual reacting by applying more pressure to the brakes unnecessarily in an effort to stop the perceived motion. This illusion can be encountered in diving in many ways, the most common of which is when diving in calm waters, where no major current or tidal movement exists to affect the diver's positioning, and when other objects like grass gently moves. The movement of the other object creates the impression that the diver themselves is moving in the opposite direction, causing them to attempt to stay in place by maneuvering their fins. This results in actually moving the diver, who then recognizes the movement, and applies a counter motion to cease this new movement, which creates another movement the diver reacts to. The cycle continues progressively moving the diver more and more out of control, and falsely leads the diver to believe they must continue to move to stay in position, whereas if they simply stopped all movements and relaxed, they'd be in more control.

(Many divers experience relative motion when other objects, especially plant life, sways in gentle currents, giving them the feeling that they themselves are moving when they're actually not.)

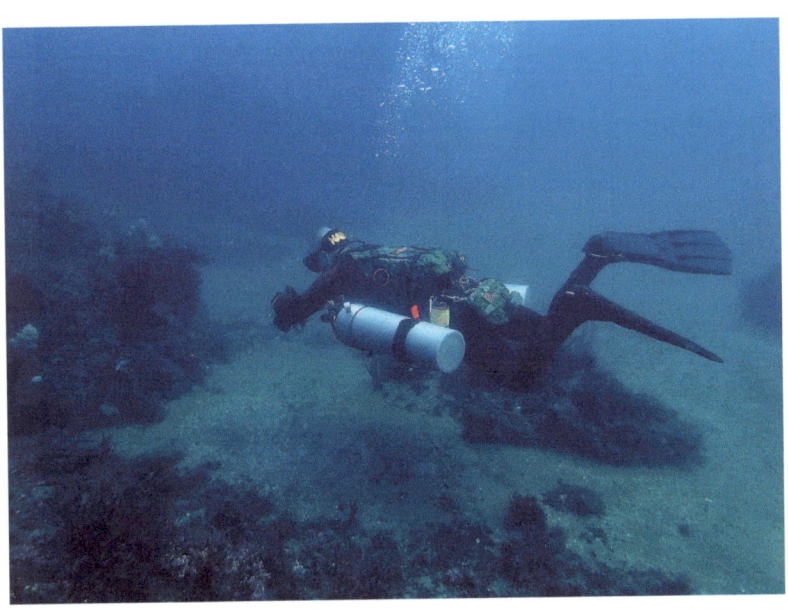

Altered Planes of Reference - Objects are so great in size (e.g. rock formation or ridge line in the distance, or the structure of a wreck you're within) that they replace the horizon. A diver can have an inaccurate sense of depth, trim attitude, or position in relation to an object, any time the object is so great in size that the object itself becomes the new plane of reference, rather than the correct horizontal plane. A diver approaching a cliff edge or large artificial structure, such as a ship wreck, may swim toward the ridgeline of the object, altering their depth unnecessarily or by mistake, causing them to dive deeper than their MOD, or ascend when they shouldn't. This is because the diver's subconscious mistakes the objects ridgeline for a horizon, which we have a natural tendency to align ourselves to. Without an adequate horizon for us to see while diving, the brain attempts to assign the object's upper-most horizontal plane as a natural horizon, which we then swim toward.

(Shipwrecks easily replace the horizontal plane due to their size.)

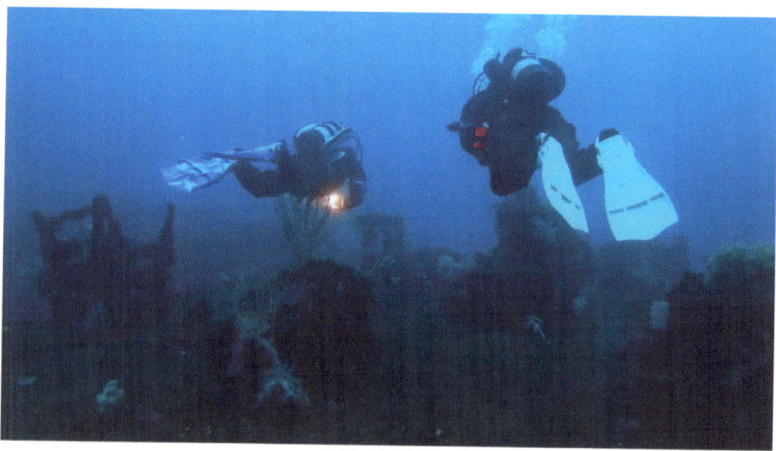

Structural Illusions - Straight lines may appear curved, and objects underwater when viewed from the surface may appear in a different location than they actually are. These illusions are caused by differences in heat, salinity, waves, rarefaction, and other visual obscurants. A straight line may appear curved or distorted when viewed through multiple layers of water with different salinity, or when one part of the water is warmer than the rest. An object may appear broken or bent when viewed entering the water from the surface or through a salinity layer, or in a different location completely if fully submerged. Objects underwater appear larger and closer than they actually are due to a rarefaction rate of 1.33, making them seem 33% larger and closer. These differences can confuse divers about the shape, actual location, and size of objects that their brain is used to seeing as a certain size.

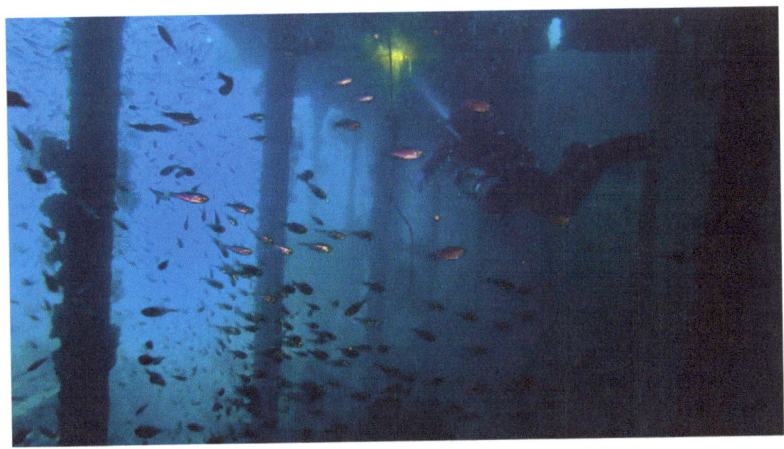

Height/Depth Perception Illusions - Lack of visual cues causes the diver to lose their depth perception. When diving in the open ocean, or an area devoid of visual references, the diver will be deprived of their perception of distance and depth. They will not be able to discern approximate distances, such as how far away a fish or object may be if it appeared within visual range, or the approximate distance to the bottom if not already known, or even the estimated actual visible range itself.

Size/Distance Illusions - Diver misinterprets objects size to be the same as what they are used to, giving them a false perception of distance from the object or reference point. This illusion most often occurs if the visual cues, such as wildlife, a rock, drop off, or artificial structure, are of a different size than initially expected. The diver may falsely believe the object is closer than it truly is if the diver expects the object to be smaller than it actually is, and vice-versa.

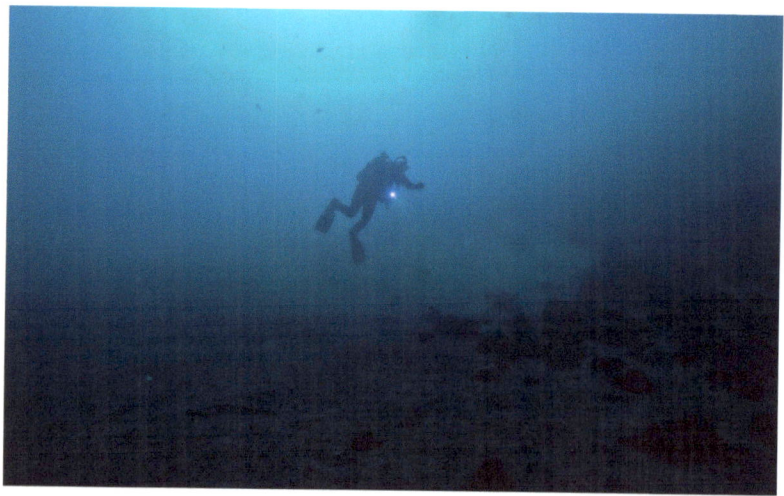

Autokinesis - Illusion of movement in which a stationary object, with no clear background, appears to move around (e.g. a black dot on a white background, or moving lines of sand amongst a sandy bottom).

Reversible Perspective - Occurs when a diver thinks an object is moving away from them, when it's actually moving toward them, and vice-versa. Usually happens at dusk or night when light is limited, or when an object is at the limit of visibility underwater, when the silhouette of the object is all that is distinguishable.

(Sometimes it can be near impossible to tell if an object is coming toward you or moving away.)

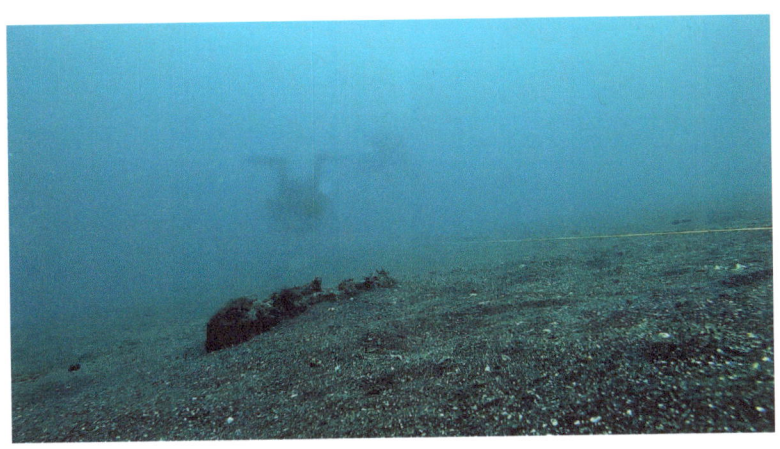

Lack of Motion Parallax - Moving nearby objects against no clear background appear to remain stationary when they should be moving opposite to the direction of travel, giving the impression you are not moving at all.

Vestibular Illusions

The vestibular system provides accurate information as long as an individual is on the ground. Once the individual is removed from the ground—either flying through the air or diving underwater—the system may function incorrectly and cause illusions that can be disorientating and even incapacitating. Vestibular illusions pose the greatest problem with spatial disorientation, and as such, it's imperative that divers understand these illusions, and the conditions under which they occur, if they are to distinguish between the inputs of the vestibular system that are accurate and those that cause illusions.

Somatogyral Illusions

Somatogyral illusions are caused when angular accelerations and decelerations stimulate the semicircular canals. Those that may be encountered when diving are the leans, graveyard spins, and the Coriolis effect.

Leans - After stabilization of the middle ear while in an unusual attitude (such as being tilted to one side), correction to the horizontal plane results in the feeling of "leaning" to the opposite side.

Graveyard Spin - After stabilization of the middle ear while in a slight turn (maintaining an unusual attitude for a prolonged period of time), correction to the horizontal plane gives the sensation of "overcorrecting" to the opposite angle, resulting in the diver re-correcting back to the previous angle and resuming the uncorrected turn. The diver thinks they are traveling in a straight line when actually they are in a continuous subtle slight turn. This can result in unintended descent or loss of navigation.

Coriolis Effect - After stabilization of the middle ear in an unusual attitude along multiple planes, sudden correction results in moving middle ear fluids along multiple planes at the same time, causing an overwhelming sensation of movement in multiple directions (extreme vertigo), and can cause incapacitation.

Somatogravic Illusions

Somatogravic illusions are caused by changes in linear accelerations and decelerations or gravity that stimulate the otolith organs. The three types of somatogravic illusions that can be encountered while diving are oculogravic, elevator, and oculoagravic.

Oculogravic Illusion - This is caused by forward acceleration, giving a sense of "high attitude" (head up, feet down trim). Diver responds by positioning themselves in a head-down trim, or through panic by deflating BC, or both. Either of which results in an unintended dive.

Elevator Illusion - Caused by upward acceleration, giving a sense of "high attitude" (head up, feet down trim). Diver responds by positioning themselves in a head-down trim, or through panic by deflating BC, or both. Either of which results in an unintended dive.

Oculoagravic Illusion - Caused by a downward acceleration (quick or rapid descent), eyes track upward and gives a sense of "low attitude" (either a head down, feet up trim, or a sense of "falling"). Diver responds by positioning themselves in a head-up trim, or through panic by inflating BC, or both. Either of which results in a premature ascent.

Proprioceptive Illusions

Proprioceptive illusions rarely occur alone. They are closely associated with the vestibular system and, to a lesser degree, with the visual system. The proprioceptive information input to the brain may also lead to a false perception of true vertical. During turns, tilts to one side or another, ascents, and descents, and the motion of the ocean, proprioceptive information is fed into the central nervous system.

A diver is exposed to gravitational forces and centrifugal forces through the movement of the body of water they are within, and without visual references, the body only senses changes in pressures and movement of internal organs. Because these sensations are normally associated with movement, the diver may falsely interpret them as such, even if the diver is not traveling in any direction.

Most new divers feel the motion of the ocean through proprioceptive inputs and falsely believe they must constantly move their body to remain in one position. They believe they are being pushed and pulled, especially in tidal areas, and have a subconscious need to apply continuous corrective actions though constant movement to control themselves in the environment, even when none may be necessary.

These actions cause further proprioceptive inputs, which leads them to make even more corrections, and thus, they themselves become the very reason they can't stay put in one place.

(Proprioceptive illusions can give us the sensation of movement, even if no movement is taking place, resulting in unconscious reactions of constant movement by the limbs in an effort to remain stationary. The ability to remain calm and relaxed, and refrain from unconscious reactions to perceived movement, is a skill all divers eventually seek to emulate, and one that takes time to develop.)

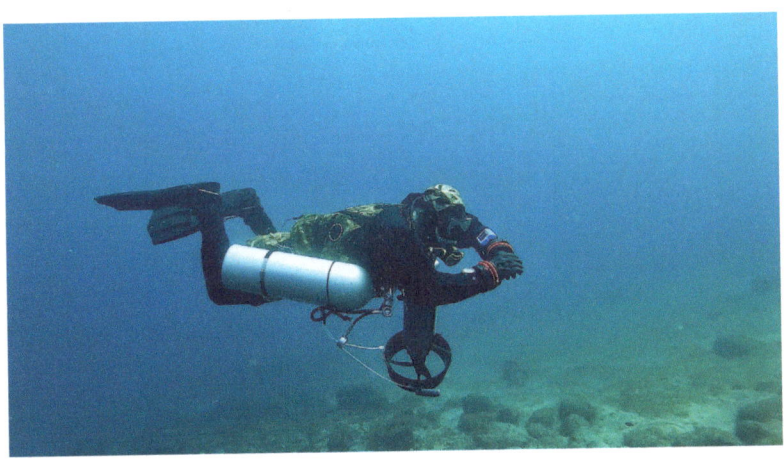

STRESS AND FATIGUE IN DIVING

Stress and fatigue in diving operations adversely affects an individual's performance, awareness, cognitive abilities, and safety. Consequently, it also shares a relationship with spatial disorientation and a diver's ability to both recognize and recover from disorientating sensory illusions. As such, divers should be familiar with the effects of stress and fatigue on the body and mind, and how their behavior and lifestyles may reduce or increase the amount of stress and fatigue they experience.

Stress

Stress is the nonspecific response of the body and mind to any demand placed upon it. Sometime around 1926, an Austrian physician named Hans Selye identified what he believed was a consistent pattern of mind-body reactions that he called "the nonspecific response of the body to any demand." He later referred to this pattern as the "rate of wear and tear on the body." In search of a term that best described these concepts, he turned to the physical sciences and borrowed the term "stress."

Selye's definition is necessarily broad because the notion of stress involves a wide range of human experiences. However, it incorporates two very important basic points: stress is a physiological phenomenon involving actual changes in the body's chemistry and function, and stress involves some perceived or actual demand for action. The definition does not qualify these demands as either positive or negative because both types of demands may be stressful. For example, although gaining a new skill for advanced diving possibilities is generally considered a positive, rewarding event, the potential ambiguity and uncertainty of the course you're about to take, and the tests you might face to earn a new certification, may be stressful.

Identifying Stressors

A stressor is any stimulus or event that requires an individual to adjust or adapt in some way—emotionally, physiologically, or behaviorally. Stressors may be psychosocial, environmental, physiological, and cognitive. Before devising an effective stress-management plan, the individual first needs to identify the significant stressors in his or her life.

Psychosocial Stressors - These are life events. These stressors may trigger adaptation or change in one's lifestyle, career, and/or interaction with others.

Job Stress - Work responsibilities can be a significant source of stress for divers. Regardless of job assignment, carrying out assigned duties often produces stress. Conflict in the workplace, low morale and cohesion, boredom, fatigue, over tasking, and poorly defined responsibilities, are all potentially debilitating job stressors. Individuals who lack confidence in their abilities, or who have problems communicating and cooperating with others, experience considerable stress.

Illness - Although divers should maintain a degree of physical fitness and health, many recreational divers see no need for fitness or a generally healthy lifestyle.

Diseases and illnesses are a source of stress, and fatigue is a common symptom of an unhealthy physical condition.

Family Issues - Although the family can be a source of emotional strength, it can also cause stress. Family commitments may adversely affect performance, particularly when concentration is high in the preparation stages of a dive. Concerns for family members or issues may become a distraction, and can increase fatigue and irritability. The potential dangers of a diver not mentally engaged in the dive may also act as a stressor on families, and may cause tension on relationships.

Environmental Stressors

Depth - The stress caused by depth is a multifaceted problem. As gasses become denser, increased work of breathing puts physical stress on the respiratory system. At the same time, with depth comes the psychological stress to perform effectively and efficiently, so as not to increase your gas consumption or the saturation of gasses in our tissues.

Hot and Cold Environments - Being physically too hot or too cold causes physical and psychological stress to divers. Waiting to get into the water on a hot summer day while fully dressed in a wetsuit or drysuit can lead to heat cramps, heat exhaustion, or even heat stroke if the diver isn't adequately hydrated or suffers too long. On the other hand, a diver without adequate thermal protection can lose core body heat fast underwater through conduction, leading to hypothermia. A diver that is too hot or too cold loses focus and suffers increasing difficulty in reaction timing and cognitive abilities.

Equipment Design - Human factors in the fitment, engineering, design, customization, weight, and comfort of equipment can significantly impact and affect individual performance. If equipment is too heavy, it could hinder a diver's ability to function and move, or even lead to injury. If the design isn't ergonomically preferable, the diver my find it difficult to use effectively, especially when necessary most.

Equipment Performance - The overall performance of each piece of equipment the diver uses can increase or decrease the stress of the diver. Poor performing regulators, bad o-rings, loose pressure release valves, loose straps, corroded latches and bolt snaps, and more, can all make a diver's life underwater miserable or worrisome. A diver focused on malfunctioning or barely functioning equipment isn't focused on the dive itself.

Time and Performance - The longer the amount of time a diver spends engrossed on a task, the more stress builds up. Additionally, stress can increase with task difficulty and if things are not going according to plan. A diver stressed about personal performance or the length to which the dive is taking, isn't effective in the water.

Social Environment - Positivity breeds positivity, while negativity loves company. If the group is unhappy, this attitude can increase stress, needlessly making the dive more difficult.

Physiological Stressors

Although divers often have limited control over a variety of aspects of diving-related stress, they can exert significant control over self-imposed stress. Many individuals engage in maladaptive behaviors that are potentially debilitating and threaten diver safety.

The memory aid for these self-imposed stressors is: **DEATH**

Drugs - All drugs, whether over the counter (OTC) or prescription, have the ability to react differently when diving. This is because increases in atmospheric pressure can alter the way chemicals react in the body. Many divers self-medicate with common-use OTC's for a range of minor ailments, to include headaches, sinus issues, and general pain management. However, most drugs, whether prescribed or OTC, have a range of potential unwanted side-effects that vary from person to person. Some side-effects can be minor, such as drowsiness or sensitivity to light, while others may be more serious, such as addiction or allergic reactions. For divers, pressure increases can also increase the potency of a drug in the diver's system, and what might be harmless on the surface, could become an overdose and fatal situation with an increase in atmospheric pressure.

Exhaustion - Tiredness reduces mental alertness. A lack of rest and proper sleep reduce performance and reaction capabilities too. In situations that require immediate actions, exhaustion causes divers to respond more slowly, if they are even capable of acknowledging the situation in a timely manner to begin with. Exhausted divers are highly susceptible to fascination/fixation. They tend to concentrate on one aspect of a situation without considering the total environment, which may lead to an emergency situation. Good physical conditioning should decrease fatigue and improve efficiency. However, excessive exercise in a short period of time can lead to increased fatigue. Multiple factors cause exhaustion, and normally, exhaustion does not set in from one factor alone. Contributing factors include poor diet habits, lack of rest, poor sleeping patterns, poor physical condition, an inadequate exercise routine, environmental factors, dehydration, and work/life stress. In combination, these can create exhaustion, and common side effects associated include altered levels of concentration, awareness, and attentiveness; increased drowsiness; and ineffective visual acuity.

Alcohol - Moderate ingestion of alcohol in the form of liquor, wine, or beer is a commonly accepted practice that usually causes no problems. For divers, however, alcohol can be deadly. Alcohol causes a person to become uncoordinated and impairs judgement, and it hinders the ability to function properly. Alcohol induces histotoxic hypoxia, which is the poisoning of the bloodstream, interfering with the use of oxygen by body tissues. Every ounce of alcohol in the bloodstream at sea level increases the body's physiological altitude. For example, one ounce of alcohol in the bloodstream at sea level places an individual at approximately 2,000 feet (610m) above sea level physiologically. Detrimental effects associated with alcohol include poor and impaired judgement, impaired decision-making, impaired perception, reduced reaction time, loss of coordination, and extreme susceptibility to fascination/fixation.

Tobacco - The detrimental effects of tobacco on health are well known. Hemoglobin in red blood cells have a 200 to 300 times greater affinity for carbon monoxide than for oxygen. That is, the hemoglobin accepts carbon monoxide far more rapidly than it will accept oxygen. During normal pulmonary perfusion (gas exchange within the lungs), carbon dioxide is released from the bloodstream when an individual exhales. When an individual inhales, the normal action is that oxygen is absorbed into the blood; thus, normal levels of oxygen and other gasses are being maintained within the body. Smoking increases CO, which in turn, reduces the capacity of the blood to carry O2. The hypoxia that results from this increase in carbon monoxide is called hypemic hypoxia, which is a reduced ability of the blood to accept and carry oxygen. Hypemic hypoxia negatively affects the peripheral vision and dark adaptation.

Hypoglycemia - Experts recognize the importance of a nutritious, well-balanced diet for divers, and it is strongly recommended to avoid missing or postponing meals. Divers should also avoid supplementing primary meals with fast sugars (candy and sodas), and high fatty foods (fast food and junk foods). These foods and beverages can cause low blood-sugar levels, which may result in hunger pangs, distraction, a breakdown in normal daily patterns, a shortened attention span, and other physiological changes. Supplementing with fast sugars as the primary diet will, on average, sustain the individual for up to 30 to 45 minutes, however, the negative effects will then increase in intensity. Poor dietary habits are also widely known to lead to diabetic conditions as constant and continuous spikes in glucose levels lead to ever-higher normalizations of insulin levels released by the pancreas to regulate the metabolism.

Cognitive Stressors

How one perceives a given situation or problem is a potentially significant and frequently overlooked source of stress. Pessimism, obsession, failure to focus on the present, and/or low self-confidence can create a self-fulfilling prophecy that will ensure a negative outcome. Albert Ellis, a renowned clinical psychologist, observed that stress results when individuals believe that things *must* go their way, or *should* conform to their own needs and desires, or they cannot function. This lack of flexibility in thinking causes problems when reality does not accommodate the individual's wishes. Failure to accept the possibility that things may happen contrary to one's wishes leaves the individual unprepared, frustrated, and dysfunctional.

Healthy individuals believe that there exist choices in life, and the more possibilities for choice, combined with the free will to exercise choice, the better. Although certain consequences may make some choices unpalatable, they are choices nonetheless. Experiencing oneself as actively making choices increases a sense of personal control and decreases stress—until it doesn't. More recent observations have shown the opposite can be true as well, that too many choices can lead some individuals to experience heightened stress levels when an inability to rule out or eliminate excessive options causes the individual to become overwhelmed. This can be especially true when a significant deadline is approaching. Unhappy, unhealthy, and overly stressed individuals often fail to see that they have choices, or maintain an inability to make a choice given an abundance of possibilities. These people have a strong tendency to see the world as the cause of all of their problems.

Finally, living in the past or the future, and overemphasizing what should have been or what could be, can increase stress. Although there is utility in both learning from the past and planning for the future, over-engaging in either can cause expel to fail at the very tasks and opportunities in the present.

Stress and Spatial Disorientation

An individual's ability to recognize and react appropriately to encountered sensory illusions and resulting spatial disorientation is greatly impacted by the degree to which stressors are affecting them during the dive, or that have been affecting them prior to the dive. An individual suffering from chronic stress prior to a dive more than likely will suffer from degraded performance during the dive, and when sensory illusions are encountered, is far less likely to be able to recognize and understand what is happening and why. Additionally, fatigued divers suffer from reduced cognitive performance, slowing their reaction timing and inhibiting their ability to make proper decisions.

Stress affects performance, and applying a range of stress management techniques to induce good stress will increase performance and produce growth. As stated prior, stress can be both good and bad, and while good stress helps you perform at peak proficiency, negative stressors ultimately impact a diver's awareness, reaction capabilities, performance, and safety. It is therefore important for divers to understand how psychological, physiological, and environmental stressors impact their their awareness and cognitive capabilities, as well as how it can directly affect their ability to react to spatial disorientation when encountered.

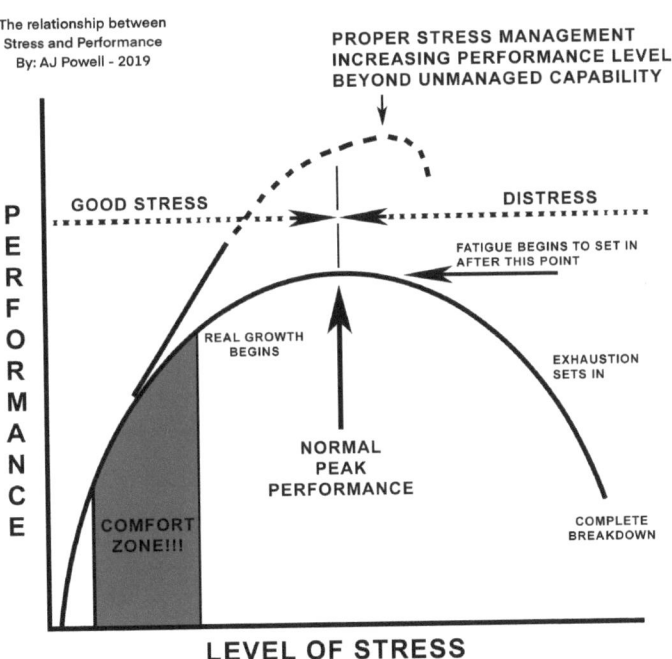

PREVENTION OF SPATIAL DISORIENTATION

Spatial disorientation can never be completely prevented due to sensory and bio-neuro conflicts. Perhaps the single most important factor is to realize that misleading sensations that come from sensory systems are predictable. Proper training, instrument proficiency, time and experience, and good health can minimize spatial disorientation, but Spatial D. becomes dangerous when divers believe their sensations rather than trusting their instruments and training.

Training

Proper training is the number one way to reduce the susceptibility to spatial disorientation. Through awareness training—whether by incorporation of spatial disorientation information into already established academic curriculum, or through a developed course of instruction on the subject alone, or through sources like this book—and practical training—such as demonstration of illusions and effects in a safe environment, and experience gained during dives over time—divers gain the ability to learn the "how's" and "why's" of how spatial disorientation occurs and affects the diver. Divers must understand the limitations of sensory mechanisms, the particular physical maneuvers and environmental factors that can produce sensations, that can lead to spatial disorientation, and the conditions where errors in perception are most likely to occur.

Additionally, a strong focus on instrument training—use and proficiency—with regards to dive computers, compasses, depth gauges, HUD's, and any other devices a diver might use to discern their position and orientation in a three dimensional space, must be performed on a regular basis in order to develop and maintain proficiency in use, and instill the mental reliance on these tools to prevent disorientation.

(Continuous training opportunities are present on every dive. A strong focus on instrument proficiency can minimize the possibilities of becoming spatially disorientated, and is especially useful when diving in environments completely void of visual cues.)

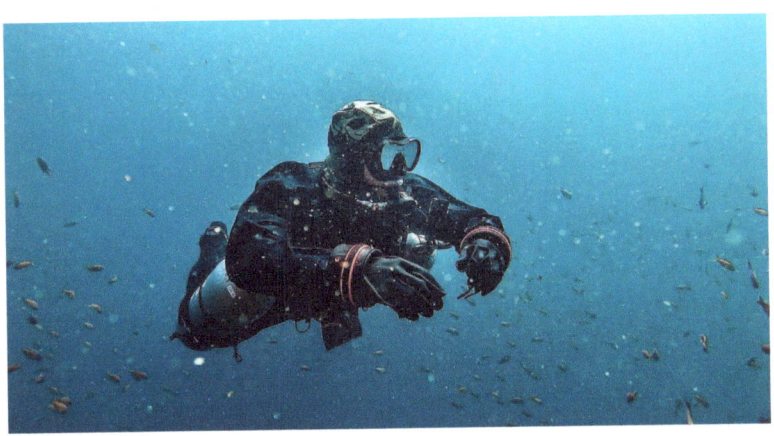

Communication and Coordination

An analysis of accidents in the aviation field revealed that significant percentages of accidents resulted from one or more crew coordination and communicational errors committed prior to the accident. Diving is no different, with a significant number of incidents every year occurring due to poor communication. Often accidents are a result of a sequence of undetected errors—either individually or as a team—that combine to produce a catastrophic result. In relation to a diver experiencing spatial disorientation, the ability to effectively communicate the problem to fellow divers may mean the difference between getting back to the surface safely or not.

Broadly defined, Communication and Coordination is the interaction between dive team members (or dive buddies) necessary for the safe, efficient, and effective execution of a planned dive, and performance of assigned tasks (if any). There exist eight Communication Elements, and five Coordination Objectives, and effective use of these can greatly aid in the prevention of spatial disorientation, as well as the ability to respond to it appropriately if encountered.

Communication Elements

Communicate Positively - Good teamwork requires positive communication. Communication is positive when the sender directs, announces, request, or offers information; the receiver follows by acknowledging the information; then the sender confirms the information was received based on the receiver's acknowledgement or action (two-challenge rule).

Direct Assistance - A diver will direct assistance when he or she cannot perform an action themselves, or when assistance is required due to the nature of the task. In emergency situations, such as a diver incapacitated by sensory illusions causing disorientation, the direction of assistance may be to provide a stabilizing hand hold, or aid the diver in reaching the surface safely.

Offer Assistance - A diver will provide assistance or information that has been requested to another diver directing assistance.

Announce Actions - To ensure effective and well-coordinated actions while on a dive, all divers should be aware of the expected movements and actions planned for the dive, as well as any individual actions if required. Each diver will announce their actions to the team or their buddy prior to initiating those actions. Doing so prevents confusion, and if any disorientation occurs thereafter, other divers will readily know and be prepared to act.

Acknowledge Actions - Communications within dive teams and between buddy pairs must include supportive feedback to ensure that members correctly understand the situation, requests, announcements, or directives.

Be Explicit - Divers should use clear signals, terms, and phrases, and positively acknowledge critical information. They must avoid using complicated signals or sets of signals, and terms that may have multiple meanings, such as "right" when they mean "correct". Additionally, signals and verbiage should avoid indefinite modifiers, such as "go up" when they mean "surface". Selecting independent, simple signals, and using specific phrases, will greatly reduce confusion and save time in communication.

Provide Advisories - Although everyone should be actively engaged in maintaining situational awareness to both their surroundings and the plan, it is not always the case that every person remembers every aspect, nor can they see every thing around them. It is therefore appropriate to provide advisories any time another diver gets too close to something they shouldn't, or may not notice a hazard, and prior to initiating the next phase of a plan.

Coordinate Action Sequences and Timing - Proper sequencing and timing of each other's actions will ensure that the actions of each diver in a team or buddy pair mesh well with the actions of the others or their buddy, as well as align properly with the intended sequence of events in the dive plan, if any.

Coordination Objectives

Establish and Maintain Relationships - All divers should work to establish Mutuility of Concern by building a positive relationship between members. Doing so allows team members the comfort and reassurance to communicate openly and freely, and to operate in a concerted manner.

Planning and Rehearsal - Divers should be willing to explore, in concert, all aspects of a dive plan, and to analyze each segment for potential difficulties and possible emergencies. Divers should never be made to feel rushed as this feeling would lead to apprehension that will carry over into the dive.

Establish and Maintain Workloads - Divers should be willing to establish, assign, and distribute work loads, and manage and execute workloads in an effective and efficient manner with redistribution of individual tasks as a situation changes.

Exchange Information - Divers should establish intra-team communications using simple and effective patterns and techniques that allow the flow of essential information between members in an easily understandable manner.

Cross-Monitor Performance - Divers should cross-monitor each other's actions, decisions, and performance, to reduce the likelihood of errors impacting proper action sequences and safety.

Response to Stress in an Emergency

Stressful situations affect individuals in a variety of ways. The most common reactions are predominantly negative in nature, and include things such as fear, anxiety, panic, apprehension, inaction, emotional outbursts, and anger. Unfortunately, these types of reactions compound problems, making stressful situations worse. For divers, this can be deadly.

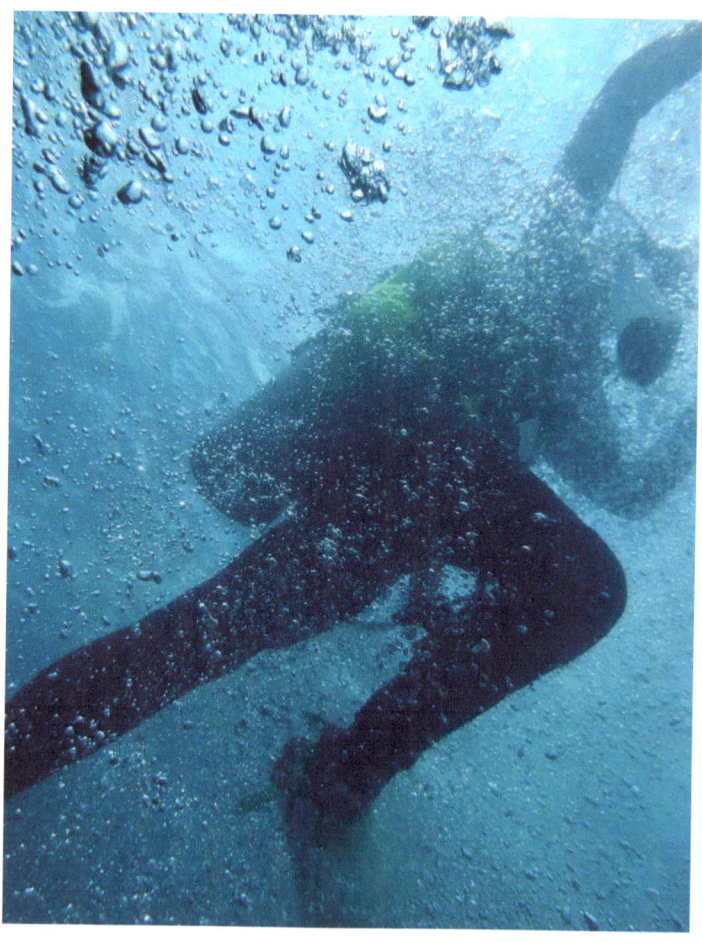

Through training and experience, most divers will become increasingly comfortable in the water and more confident in their Knowledge, Skills, and Abilities (KSA's). A diver's growth allows them to react more appropriately to any given unexpected situation encountered underwater. Often times, what seems like an emergency really isn't, and if a diver becomes disorientated underwater, it does not necessarily constitute an emergency. The best behavioral response is to remain calm and focus on breathing. Next would be to understand that the immediate action they may instinctively want to take might not be the best decision to make. Therefore, delaying these intuitive actions, and instead, focusing on identifying the problem, and its associated resolutions, would be the next best possible course of action.

Divers should be cautions of developing Stress-Related Regression, whereby individuals under stressful conditions will forget learned procedures and skill, causing them to instinctually revert to bad habits. They should also be mindful of Perceptual Tunneling, a phenomenon in which an individual, or even an entire team under stress, becomes focused on one stimulus. Most sensory illusions will resolve themselves in a short period of time given that no biological emergency exists that is causing them, or that some environmental factor exists perpetuating them. If the diver experiencing disorientation establishes a stabilizing hold on a stationary object, or receives the assistance of another diver, remains calm, and thinks through the problem, they may find the effects likely to subside and resolve themselves, leaving them able to carry on with the dive without incident.

TREATMENT OF SPATIAL DISORIENTATION

The process by which spatial disorientation is treated is relatively simple. That being said, a diver actively experiencing severe sensory illusions causing extreme disorientation may be likely to panic. The ability to handle such a situation isn't a universal development either. It's not as if time and experience are the only factors determining whether or not any one particular individual will respond to such stress in a safe way. There are many individuals who have over a thousand logged dives, and hundreds of hours accumulated underwater, and yet they may never have encountered a severe problem likely to induce panic. Therefore, it is essential for divers to understand that each encounter with sensory illusions may be unique and situationally dependent, however, the proper reaction to each case of spatial disorientation generally remains the same.

REMAIN CALM and breath

Above all else, if you only do one thing, remain calm. Remember that what you're experiencing is the result of sensory illusions. Though the world may appear to be spinning, or you may feel like you're leaning, or even if you're nauseous and dizzy, if you panic, you will turn a non-emergency into an actual emergency. You have air, so you're not going to drown. Remain calm and breath normally, and you very well may find that this simple first step gives just the time needed for the effects to resolve themselves.

Delay Intuitive Action(s)

Most new diver's instinctual actions any time something goes wrong or makes them feel uncomfortable is to bolt for the surface. If they don't do that, next, primacy will have a strong tendency to cause the diver to move their body into a posture typically experienced during training. If divers were trained on their knees—the worst thing an instructor can do to set the student up for future hardship—they will instinctively "go to their knees" any time they become stressed to begin addressing the problem. Going to your knees alters your buoyancy characteristics, causing you to sink, or if you're kicking, causing you to prematurely surface. Either of which turns a non-emergency into a potential emergency as the problem is compounded by additional new dilemmas the diver must deal with. The best response is to take no response at all. Stop moving, don't alter your posture, and give yourself time to understand what is happening before making any changes.

Communicate Problem (if able)

Divers should not attempt to handle problems by themselves if they are diving with a team or as a buddy pair. Even if disorientated, most people are still able to communicate simple messages to some degree in order to ask for help and establish that a problem exists. Clear, simplistic communication can effectively get the message across to others that you need assistance. Whether it's help in stabilizing yourself, or getting to the surface, don't go at it alone.

Rely on Instruments and Cues

You may "feel" like you're moving or tilted or turning or that you're someplace you may not be, but while your senses will lie to you, your instruments will not. Your compass can do more than merely tell you direction. It also tilts inside the case, and can tell you if you are tilted in an altered plane of reference too. You may feel as if you're changing depth due to relative motion, but your computer or depth gauge will verify if that feeling is true or false. How do you know if your trim attitude is off after your middle ear has stabilized to a false horizon prior to exiting a wreck? Bubbles always go "up", and you can use this cue to determine the proper X and Y axis in relation to the true horizon. Relying on your instruments and monocular cues will aid you in problem-solving and dealing with spatial disorientation when encountered.

Slow Down/Think Through Problem

Real emergencies have "immediate actions" that all divers should know, be trained to perform, and practice regularly to carry out. Spatial disorientation, however, is rarely an emergency. The only time spatial disorientation becomes an emergency, is if the sensory illusions encountered are severe enough to incapacitate the affected diver. Examples can include the Coriolis effect, and seizures induced from flicker vertigo, just to name two possibilities. Most cases of spatial disorientation are not actual emergencies, and if you simply slow down and think, you'll likely find an easy resolution exists, or that the problem goes away, leaving you able to move on and continue the dive.

Anchor Yourself

Many sensory illusions exist due to conflicts between what we see and feel, and most of the time, these can be resolved by grabbing hold of a nearby object anchored in place—such as a rock or other large, heavy object—or by holding onto another diver. Motion sickness can work this way, as can dizziness caused by vestibular illusions. Once we hold on to something that anchors us in place, most will find the effects of these sensory illusions dissipate, and they are able to carry on with the dive thereafter.

Remember, if you become spatially disorientated due to encountering sensory illusions while underwater, above all else, remain calm, breath, delay intuitive actions, try to communicate the problem, check your instruments, grab something, and try to work through the problem if able until it subsides.

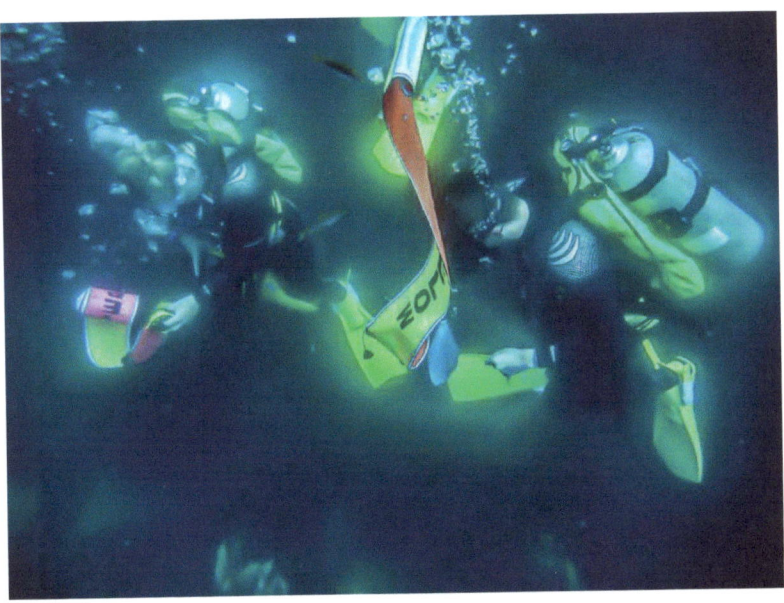

/// THIS PAGE INTENTIONALLY LEFT BLANK ///

/// THIS PAGE INTENTIONALLY LEFT BLANK ///

Appendix

Common Terms and Definitions

Astigmatism: An unequal curvature of the cornea or lens of the eye.

Attitude: The pitch and trim of an object in relation to the horizontal plane.

BC: Buoyancy Compensator.

CCR: Closed-Circuit Rebreather.

Chronic: A continued or prolonged condition; for example, a chronic illness continuing for several years.

Endolymph: The watery fluid contained in the membranous labyrinth of the ear.

Fatigue: Term used to describe an overall feeling of tiredness or a lack of energy.

FoV: Field-of-View.

Ghost Sensations: Memories of sensations the individual continues to feel for a period of time as if they were still occurring, despite that the actual sensations have ceased.

Heat Cramps: A condition marked by sudden development of cramps in skeletal muscles, resulting from prolonged exposure to high temperatures and accompanied by profuse perspiration with loss of sodium chloride (salt) from the body.

Heat Exhaustion: A condition marked by weakness, nausea, dizziness, and profuse sweating, resulting from prolonged physical exertion in a hot environment.

Heat Stroke: An abnormal physiological condition produced by exposure to intense heat and characterized by hot, dry skin, vomiting, convulsions, and collapse, in which severe cases can be fatal.

HUD: Heads-Up-Display.

Hyperopia: A refraction error in which the lens of the eye does not focus an image directly on the retina, but behind it instead, causing far-sightedness.

Hypothermia: A loss of core body heat, at a rate faster than the body can generate heat, characterized by shivering, low body temperature, and blueness of the skin in mild cases, and mental confusion, no shivering, and tiredness in extreme cases.

Hypoxia: A lack of oxygen condition in the body. There exist four types of hypoxia: Hypoxic Hypoxia (general condition of overall lack of oxygen), Hypemic Hypoxia (a reduction in the oxygen-carrying capacity of the blood, also called "anemic hypoxia), Stagnant Hypoxia (inadequate circulation of the blood preventing oxygenation of the body), and Histotoxic

Hypoxia (interference with the body's ability to absorb O2 - alcohol, drugs, etc.).

<u>Iodopsin:</u> The photosensitive chemical that is always present in cone photoreceptor cells that allows the eye to perceive light, color, clarity and detail.

<u>KSA's:</u> Knowledge, Skills and Abilities.

<u>Mesopic Vision:</u> Vision used in transition lighting such as dawn and dusk conditions.

<u>MOD:</u> Maximum Operating Depth.

<u>Monocular Cues:</u> Visual cues used to determine distance and size estimation of objects.

<u>Mutuility of Concern:</u> The degree to which individual members of a team or group see themselves as an important and valued member of that team or group.

<u>Myopia:</u> An refraction error in which the lens of the eye does not focus an image directly onto the retina, but before it instead, causes near-sightedness.

<u>Night Myopia:</u> Myopia induced by blue wavelengths of light prevalent in the visible portion of the spectrum.

<u>OTC:</u> Over-the-Counter.

<u>Otolith Organs:</u> Small sacs located in the vestibule that contains chalk-like crystals, called otoliths, which respond to gravity and linear acceleration/deceleration.

Photopic Vision: Daytime vision, characterized by full color vision capable of seeing details.

Presbyopia: The normal aging process of the eye, which causes the lens of the eye to harden.

Retinal Rivalry: Both eyes simultaneously attempting to perceive two dissimilar objects independently, resulting in one eye dominating the other.

Semicircular Canals: Three perpendicular canals, filled with a fluid called endolymph, that respond to angular acceleration changes along the X, Y, and Z axis's (pitch, roll, and yaw attitudes).

Scotopic Vision: Vision used at night and in limited lighting conditions, characterized by black and white, and shades of gray only, peripheral vision.
Rarefaction: The reduction in density of an object or wave (e.g. light). The opposite of compression.

Rhodopsin: The photosensitive chemical produced by rod photoreceptor cells that allows the eye to detect far lower levels of light necessary for night vision.

Sensory Illusion: A sensory illusion is a false perception of reality caused by the conflict of orientation information from one or more mechanisms of equilibrium. Sensory illusions are a major cause of Spatial D.

Spatial Disorientation (Spatial D.): An individual's inability to determine his or her position, attitude, and motion relative to the space they are occupying and/or any significant objects within visual range.

Stress: The nonspecific response of the body and mind to any demand placed upon them.

Target Fixation: A term used to describe a diver so intensely focus on one object or goal, that they ignore other, more important information or cues that my help them solve the problem or accomplish the task, or fail to recognize that more important problems or tasks need attention rather than the one they are focused on. Also known as "perceptual tunneling" and "target hypnosis".

Task Saturation: A term used to describe an individual so overwhelmed by one or more tasks or problems that they lose the ability to manage them effectively. Also known as "task loading".

True Horizon: The natural horizontal plane of the earth by which we are biologically adapted to aligning ourselves to.

Vertigo: Vertigo is a spinning sensation usually caused by a peripheral vestibular abnormality in the middle ear. Divers and aviators alike often misuse the term vertigo, applying it generically to all forms of Spatial D. or dizziness.

Sensory Illusions: Illusions caused by false impressions or misconceptions of actual conditions created whenever a conflict exists between the input information by sensory organs and the brains interpretation of that information.

Spatial Disorientation for Divers
AJ Powell (USA, Ret.)
Copyright © 2022
All rights reserved.

All diving images within this publication are original images taken by and owned by AJ Powell, and copyright © is retained by the owner.

www.ingramcontent.com/pod-product-compliance
Lightning Source LLC
Chambersburg PA
CBHW042048290426
44109CB00006B/144